POTS SYNDROME DIET COOKBOOK

Delicious, Nutrient-Rich Recipes, Meal Plans And Guidelines To Manage Symptoms, Boost Energy, Improve Heart Health And More – All You Need To Know

DR. AMARI VALERIE

TABLE OF CONTENTS

BONUS:

7 days meal plan recipes, ingredients, and detailed preparatory guidelines for POTS Syndrome

7 Desserts procedural recipes for POTS Syndrome and guidelines

7 Smoothies procedural recipes for POTS Syndrome and guidelines

DISCLAIMER

The information provided in this book, is for educational and informational purposes only and is not intended as medical advice. The content is not a substitute for professional medical advice, diagnosis, or treatment. Always seek the advice of your physician or other qualified health provider with any questions you may have regarding a medical condition. Never disregard professional medical advice or delay in seeking it because of something you have read in this book.

The dietary suggestions and recipes in this book are based on general guidelines and may not be suitable for everyone. Individual responses to foods can vary, and it is important to consult with a healthcare professional before making any significant changes to your diet.

The author and publisher of this book do not claim to cure or treat any medical condition. The information provided is based on research and personal experience and is intended to help readers make informed decisions about their diet and health.

Furthermore, I the author do not endorse any specific products, brands, treatments, or services that may be mentioned in this book. Any references to products, services, websites, or organizations are provided for informational purposes only and do not constitute an endorsement or recommendation by the author. The inclusion of such references does not imply any association, sponsorship, or affiliation between the author and the referenced entities.

The recipes and dietary suggestions in this book are designed to be safe and healthful. However, readers should use their own discretion and consult with a healthcare professional when necessary, especially if they have allergies, sensitivities, or other dietary restrictions.

By using this book, you acknowledge and agree that the author and publisher shall not be held liable for any loss or damage, including but not limited to special, incidental, consequential, or other damages, resulting from the use of the information and recipes contained in this book.

ABOUT THIS BOOK

This "POTS Syndrome Diet Cookbook" is an indispensable resource for those who are affected by Postural Orthostatic Tachycardia Syndrome (POTS). This book commences with a comprehensive introduction that offers a detailed comprehension of POTS, including its definition, prevalent symptoms, and their impact on daily life. It emphasizes the critical role of diet in the management of POTS, as it emphasizes the necessity of a nutrient-rich diet to alleviate symptoms and enhance the overall quality of life. The introduction also provides a concise summary of this book's content, thereby preparing readers for the upcoming voyage.

This book explores the science behind POTS and nutrition, demonstrating the direct correlation between diet and POTS symptoms. It addresses the significance of maintaining blood volume and appropriate circulation through balanced meals, the relationship between POTS and hydration, and the key nutrients that are essential for managing POTS. This section establishes a scientific foundation that enables readers to comprehend the importance of a meticulously planned diet in the management of their condition.

The grocery purchasing and meal prep suggestions section is replete with practical advice. In this section, readers will discover advice on the importance of incorporating fresh, whole foods into their diet, as well as guidance on creating a POTS-friendly grocery list and meal planning and preparation techniques. It also provides budget-friendly purchasing strategies and recommendations for time-saving household gadgets and tools, thereby making healthy dining accessible and manageable.

Essential kitchen equipment and tools, fundamental cooking techniques, and secure food handling practices are all addressed in this book, which is designed for individuals who are new to cooking. It also offers advice on how to read and comprehend recipes, as well as how to modify them to accommodate specific dietary requirements. This guarantees that even novices can confidently prepare nutritious dishes.

This comprehensive guide addresses common concerns and frequently asked questions, providing solutions for managing food sensitivities and allergies, dining out with POTS, and managing flare-ups. This book also addresses critical inquiries regarding the potential advantages of supplements for individuals with POTS and their sodium intake.

This cookbook's core is its comprehensive chapters on a variety of meal types, which commence with the fundamentals of a POTS-friendly diet. It provides a comprehensive overview of the fundamental dietary principles, the significance of hydration and electrolytes, the foods and beverages that are recommended, and those that should be avoided.

Additionally, it includes a sample daily meal plan. The subsequent chapters offer a variety of recipes, including nutrient-dense breakfast options, energizing lunch ideas, gratifying supper recipes, and easy-to-make snacks and small morsels. Each recipe is intended to be both palatable and conducive to a diet that is suitable for individuals with POTS.

Hydration is essential for the management of POTS, and this book contains a chapter that is specifically dedicated to beverage preparations and hydration. This book discusses the significance of maintaining hydration, provides recipes for electrolyte-rich beverages, and investigates the advantages of herbal teas, smoothies, and infused water.

This book provides readers with comprehensive meal planning and preparation strategies to assist them in incorporating these dietary adjustments into their lives. It encompasses advice on the organization of the kitchen for efficiency, bulk cooking and preserving, and the development of a weekly meal plan. This book includes detailed recipes and guidelines for a 7-day meal plan, desserts, and smoothies that are specifically designed for POTS, and sample meal plans that accommodate a variety of requirements.

Finally, this book delves into the more comprehensive aspects of thriving with POTS, providing lifestyle advice that encompasses the significance of sleep and rest, stress management techniques, safe exercise practices, and the establishment of a supportive network. It also underscores the significance of monitoring and documenting progress, which assists readers in maintaining motivation and updating them on their progress toward improved health.

CHAPTER ONE

Comprehending Pots Syndrome

A disorder of the autonomic nervous system that predominantly impacts the regulation of blood flow is Postural Orthostatic Tachycardia Syndrome (POTS). It is distinguished by a sudden rise in heart rate upon standing, which results in symptoms such as fatigue, vertigo, syncope, and lightheadedness. These symptoms frequently cause individuals with POTS to experience difficulty with daily activities, which can have a substantial effect on their quality of life.

The Importance Of Diet In The Management Of POTS

Diet is essential for the management of POTS symptoms and the enhancement of overall well-being. A diet that is nutrient-rich and well-balanced can assist in the optimization of energy levels, the reduction of inflammation, and the stabilization of blood pressure. Key dietary strategies for managing POTS include avoiding triggers such as caffeine and alcohol, which can exacerbate symptoms, consuming small, frequent meals to prevent blood sugar fluctuations, and increasing fluid and sodium intake to improve blood volume and hydration.

The Significance Of A Nutrient-Rich Diet

To effectively manage symptoms and maintain overall health, individuals with POTS must consume a diet that is abundant in nutrients. This diet should consist of a diverse selection of whole foods that are high in fiber, antioxidants, vitamins, and minerals.

Fruits, vegetables, fruits, lean proteins, whole cereals, nuts, seeds, and healthy lipids are all examples of nutrient-rich foods that are beneficial for POTS patients. These foods are essential for the provision of nutrients that support cardiovascular health, immune function, and energy production, thereby alleviating POTS symptoms and enhancing quality of life.

The Effects Of Common Symptoms On Daily Life

Common symptoms of POTS, including fatigue, vertigo, and palpitations, can have a substantial impact on daily life and make even the most basic tasks difficult.

For instance, individuals with POTS may encounter challenges standing for extended periods, struggle to conc5entrate or complete tasks due to brain confusion, and have insufficient stamina for physical activities.

These symptoms can result in frustration and a loss of independence, as they can disrupt work, school, social activities, and overall quality of life.

A Definition And Overview Of POTS Syndrome

Postural Orthostatic Tachycardia Syndrome (POTS) is a dysautonomia that is distinguished by an excessive increase in heart rate during the transition from a lie-down to a standing position. Dizziness, lightheadedness, syncope, fatigue, vertigo, and sweating are indicators of this rapid heart rate (tachycardia).

Effectively managing symptoms through lifestyle modifications, such as dietary adjustments, is crucial for individuals with POTS, as it can significantly affect daily life and function.

The Scientific Basis Of POTS And Nutrition

Postural Orthostatic Tachycardia Syndrome (POTS) is a condition characterized by a malfunction of the autonomic nervous system, which results in symptoms such as fatigue, vertigo, and a rapid pulse rate when standing. The management of POTS symptoms is significantly influenced by nutrition, as specific foods can affect energy levels, blood flow, and overall well-being.

For example, foods that are high in sodium can contribute to the increase in blood volume, which is frequently deficient in POTS patients as a result of blood accumulating in the lower extremities. Furthermore, the prevention of blood sugar fluctuations, which can exacerbate symptoms, can be achieved through the consumption of small, frequent meals.

Influence of Diet on POTS Symptoms: The nutrients we consume can directly affect POTS symptoms. For instance, meals that are high in carbohydrates and sugar can result in blood sugar fluctuations and falls, which can exacerbate fatigue and vertigo.

Conversely, meals that are well-balanced and consist of a variety of fruits and vegetables, complex carbohydrates, lean proteins, and healthy lipids, offer steady energy and promote overall health.

It is also crucial to restrict caffeine and alcohol consumption, as they can exacerbate symptoms such as vertigo and palpitations and dehydrate the body.

Key Nutrients for POTS Management: Numerous nutrients are crucial for the management of POTS symptoms.

Symptoms such as vertigo and lightheadedness can be alleviated by increasing sodium intake, which can help expand blood volume and improve circulation.

Bananas, asparagus, and sweet potatoes are examples of potassium-rich foods that can assist in the regulation of blood pressure and resistance to muscle lethargy.

Magnesium is an additional essential nutrient that promotes the proper functioning of muscles and nerves, thereby alleviating symptoms such as muscle spasms and fatigue.

The Connection Between Hydration and POTS: It is essential to maintain proper hydration to effectively manage POTS symptoms, as dehydration can exacerbate symptoms such as fatigue, vertigo, and cognitive fog.

Drinking an adequate quantity of water throughout the day is beneficial for cardiovascular function and blood volume maintenance. Nevertheless, it may not be sufficient for POTS patients to merely increase their water intake. Consuming electrolyte-rich beverages, such as coconut water or sports drinks, can assist in the replenishment of electrolytes that have been lost through excessive perspiration or urinary output.

Comprehension of Blood Volume and Circulation: Patients with POTS frequently experience symptoms such as fatigue and vertigo as a result of low blood volume and impaired circulation.

Consuming foods that are high in iron, such as poultry, red meat, and lentils, can enhance the delivery of oxygen to tissues and promote the production of healthy blood.

Furthermore, the assimilation of iron can be improved by consuming foods that are high in vitamin C, such as bell peppers and citrus fruits.

Additionally, the consumption of foods that are abundant in vitamin B12, such as fish, eggs, and dairy products, is advantageous, as it promotes the production of red blood cells and neurological function.

CHAPTER TWO

Tips For Grocery Shopping And Meal Preparation

When purchasing a diet that is compatible with POTS, prioritize fresh, whole foods that are abundant in vitamins, minerals, and electrolytes. Include an abundance of fruits, vegetables, lean proteins, and whole grains in your grocery list. Select low-sodium alternatives to facilitate fluid retention. Divide your purchases into portions for convenient access throughout the week when meal preparation.

Invest in reusable containers to store pre-prepared meals and refreshments. For hands-off cookery, it is advisable to employ a slow cooker or Instant Pot, which can save you both time and energy. Foods that are easily digestible and do not exacerbate symptoms should be prioritized.

To assist in the regulation of blood pressure and hydration levels, prioritize foods that are high in potassium, magnesium, and water content when creating your grocery list. Avocados, mangoes, sweet potatoes, salmon, and leafy vegetables should be incorporated.

To prevent fluid retention, opt for low-sodium alternatives, including unsalted almonds, poultry, and raw meats. Remember to replenish your supply of electrolyte-rich beverages and coconut water, which are indispensable for maintaining proper hydration.

Incorporate herbs and seasonings to enhance the flavor of your dish without the need for excessive sodium.

Plan your meals to ensure that you have a steady supply of energy throughout the day by incorporating a variety of nutritious lipids, carbohydrates, and protein. Rice, quinoa, and roasted vegetables are prepared in bulk to serve as the foundation for a variety of dishes. Fruits and vegetables that have been pre-cut are ideal for incorporating into salads or stir-fries for a fast refreshment.

Utilize a variety of culinary techniques, including steaming, baking, or barbecuing, to maintain the appeal of your meals. To prevent symptoms from exacerbating, it is important to exercise portion control. For personalized meal planning advice, it is advisable to consult with a registered dietitian.

Fresh, whole foods are indispensable for the management of POTS symptoms, as they supply essential nutrients that promote overall health and well-being. These foods are inherently abundant in antioxidants, minerals, and vitamins, which can aid in the reduction of inflammation and the preservation of heart health.

The optimal health of an individual is promoted by the inclusion of a diverse array of nutrients, which is achieved by incorporating a diversity of colorful fruits and vegetables. Brown rice and cereals are examples of whole grains that offer a consistent release of energy, thereby preventing blood sugar fluctuations and collapses. You can enhance your nutrition and more effectively manage POTS symptoms by prioritizing fresh, whole foods.

Strategies For Purchasing That Are Cost-Effective:

To adhere to a budget while purchasing a POTS-friendly diet, it is important to prioritize cost-effective essentials such as frozen fruits and vegetables, lentils, and beans. When feasible, purchase in quantity to capitalize on discounts and minimize waste. To save money without compromising quality, seek out sales and coupons for items such as whole grains and lean proteins.

Shop at discount grocers or purchase store-brand products to ensure that your budget is expanded. Impulse purchases and expenditures can also be prevented through meal planning and adhering to a purchasing list. By employing strategic purchasing and meticulous planning, it is feasible to sustain a nutritious diet while adhering to financial constraints.

Fundamentals Of Cooking For Novices

It may appear to be an overwhelming task to begin preparing, but it is much easier than it appears. To begin, become acquainted with fundamental kitchen equipment and tools, including blades, cutting boards, pots, pans, and measuring containers.

Learn essential culinary techniques like sautéing, simmering, and baking. To prevent foodborne illnesses, it is important to adhere to safe food handling practices, including cleaning hands before and after handling food, separating fresh meats from other ingredients, and cooking food to the appropriate internal temperature.

As you develop your confidence, begin to experiment with the process of reading and comprehending recipes, following the step-by-step instructions to prepare delectable meals.

Do not hesitate to modify recipes to accommodate your dietary requirements or preferences by substituting ingredients or modifying portion sizes.

Kitchen Tools And Equipment That Are Essential

Providing your kitchen with the necessary instruments can enhance the efficiency and enjoyment of preparation. Begin by acquiring fundamental kitchenware, including a chef's knife, cutting board, mixing basins, measuring cups and utensils, and a collection of pots and pans of varying sizes.

Invest in high-quality tools that will endure, such as a non-stick skillet for effortless cooking and cleaning, and a durable blender or food processor for blending sauces and stews. Possessing the appropriate apparatus will enable you to confidently attempt any recipe.

Fundamental Cooking Methods

The key to preparing delectable dishes is to master basic culinary techniques. Learn how to sauté vegetables to enhance their flavor, boil pasta until it is al dente for the ideal texture, and broil meats and vegetables for a crusty exterior and tender interior.

Discover your preferred flavors and textures by experimenting with various culinary methods. As you continue to practice, you will develop a greater sense of confidence in the kitchen and be able to successfully navigate more intricate recipes.

Safe Food Handling Procedures

It is imperative to adhere to safe food handling practices to guarantee the safety of your meals and prevent the transmission of contaminated illnesses. Before and after handling food, particularly raw proteins, ensure that your hands are thoroughly washed with detergent and water. To prevent cross-contamination, it is important to keep raw meats separate from other ingredients. Additionally, it is recommended to use separate cutting surfaces and utensils for meat and produce.

Use a food thermometer to cook food to the appropriate internal temperature and promptly refrigerate any remnants to prevent spoilage. By adhering to these guidelines, you can savor your meals with tranquility.

Comprehending And Reading Recipes

It is crucial to be able to read and comprehend recipes, as they are akin to roadmaps that direct you through the culinary process. To familiarize yourself with the ingredients and procedures, begin by reading the entire recipe from beginning to end.

Be mindful of the culinary times and temperatures, as well as any specialized apparatus or techniques that may be necessary. Divide the recipe into manageable phases and collect all the essential ingredients before commencing. If you come across unfamiliar terms or ingredients, do not hesitate to google them or request clarification. As you continue to practice, you will develop a greater sense of assurance in your capacity to adhere to recipes and prepare delectable meals.

CHAPTER THREE

Frequently Asked Questions And Common Concerns

There are a multitude of inquiries and concerns that can arise when one is living with Postural Orthostatic Tachycardia Syndrome (POTS). It is not uncommon to contemplate lifestyle modifications, dietary modifications, and symptom management.

Inquiries regarding symptoms, triggers, and treatment options are frequently sought. Some individuals may question the efficacy of different lifestyle interventions or the function of diet in managing POTS symptoms.

By addressing these prevalent concerns, individuals with POTS can more effectively manage their condition and feel more empowered.

It is imperative to identify and effectively manage food sensitivities and allergies, as they can exacerbate symptoms of POTS. Maintaining a food diary to monitor symptoms following meals can assist in identifying potential triggers.

The identification of specific triggers can be facilitated by elimination diets, which involve the temporary removal of common allergens such as dairy, gluten, and soy, followed by a systematic reintroduction.

Furthermore, the risk of triggering symptoms can be reduced by selecting whole, unprocessed foods and avoiding artificial additives. Personalized guidance in effectively managing food sensitivities and allergies can be obtained by consulting with a healthcare provider or registered dietitian who specializes in POTS.

Dining out with POTS can be challenging; however, it is feasible to relish meals outside the home while reducing symptom flare-ups with adequate preparation and planning. Opt for restaurants that provide customizable or made-to-order dishes, which enable you to have more control over the size of the portions and the ingredients.

 It is also beneficial to examine the menu online in advance to identify options that are compatible with POTS. Request modifications during the ordering process, such as steamed vegetables in place of fried, dressing on the side, or substitutions for trigger foods. While effectively managing POTS symptoms, it is possible to ensure a more pleasurable dining experience by communicating dietary needs and preferences to restaurant staff.

Comprehending And Overcoming Flare-Ups
Individuals with POTS may experience flare-ups, which are periods of heightened symptoms that can occur without warning. It is possible to reduce the frequency and severity of flare-ups by comprehending common triggers, including dehydration, humidity, tension, and specific foods. Empowering individuals to regain control during exacerbations can be achieved by creating a personalized flare-up management plan that may involve lifestyle modifications, relaxation techniques, and pharmaceutical adjustments.

To effectively manage flare-ups and prevent them from interfering with daily life, it is crucial to prioritize self-care, heed to the body's signals, and seek support from healthcare professionals or support groups when necessary.

Salt And POTS: What Is The Appropriate Quantity?

Salt consumption is essential for the management of POTS symptoms, as it enhances orthostatic tolerance and increases blood volume. Depending on the specific requirements of the individual and the recommendations of their healthcare provider, the recommended daily sodium intake for individuals with POTS can vary, but it typically falls within the range of 2,500 to 5,000 milligrams or more.

To prevent potential adverse effects such as hypertension or bloating, it is crucial to ingest sodium strategically throughout the day, rather than all at once.

Salty treats, electrolyte-rich beverages, or the addition of salt to meals can assist in the maintenance of adequate sodium levels and the relief of hypovolemia symptoms, which are a prevalent concern in POTS.

FAQ: Are Supplements Effective For POTS?

Although dietary supplements may be beneficial in conjunction with a POTS management plan, they should be implemented with caution and under the supervision of a healthcare provider. Electrolytes, such as magnesium and potassium, as well as vitamins D and B12, are frequently employed in the management of POTS.

The efficacy of these supplements may vary among individuals, but they may assist in addressing nutritional deficiencies or supporting cardiovascular function.

It is imperative to consult with a healthcare provider before using any new supplements, as specific formulations or concentrations may interact with medications or exacerbate preexisting symptoms.

Furthermore, it is essential to prioritize a balanced diet that is abundant in whole foods, with supplements functioning as a supplementary measure rather than a primary treatment for POTS symptoms.

CHAPTER FOUR

The Fundamentals Of A POTS-Friendly Diet

A POTS-friendly diet is characterized by the prevention of stimuli that can exacerbate symptoms and the maintenance of stable blood sugar levels. This entails ingesting small, frequent meals throughout the day to prevent blood pressure drops that may occur after dining.

To ensure that sustained energy is provided without causing blood sugar surges or collapses, meals should be composed of a balanced combination of carbohydrates, proteins, and healthy fats.

Key Dietary Principles for POTS: The key principles of a POTS-friendly diet include limiting caffeine and alcohol consumption, increasing sodium intake to expand blood volume and improve circulation, and avoiding processed foods rich in sugar and refined carbohydrates. Furthermore, individuals with POTS should endeavor to consume foods that are abundant in vitamins and minerals to promote their overall health and well-being.

Hydration and electrolytes are essential for individuals with POTS to prevent dehydration, which can exacerbate symptoms such as fatigue and vertigo. It is imperative to consume an adequate quantity of water throughout the day, and the addition of electrolytes, such as sodium and potassium, to beverages can assist in the preservation of appropriate fluid balance and the preservation of cardiovascular function.

Recommended Foods and Beverages: Lean proteins, such as chicken, fish, and tofu, as well as complex carbohydrates like whole cereals and fruits, and healthy lipids from sources such as avocados and nuts, are all recommended for a POTS-friendly diet.

Essential vitamins and minerals are obtained by consuming an abundance of fruits and vegetables, while calcium intake can be supplemented with dairy or non-dairy alternatives. Water with electrolytes and herbal infusions are optimal beverage options.

Foods and Beverages to Avoid: Individuals with POTS should refrain from consuming foods and beverages that can exacerbate symptoms, such as high-sodium processed foods, sweetened munchies and beverages, caffeine, and alcohol. These substances have the potential to exacerbate orthostatic intolerance and other symptoms of POTS by causing dehydration, blood pressure fluctuations, and an elevated pulse rate.

Typical Daily Meal Plan: A typical daily meal plan for an individual with POTS might include a breakfast of oatmeal with berries and almond butter, a mid-morning snack of Greek yogurt with honey, a lunch of a turkey and avocado wrap with whole-grain bread, an afternoon snack of carrot sticks with hummus, and a dinner of grilled salmon with quinoa and roasted vegetables. It is crucial to maintain hydration by consuming herbal tea or water with electrolytes throughout the day.

Breakfast Recipes To Kickstart Your Day

Smoothie Recipes That Are Rich In Nutrients:

Begin your day with a protein-rich smoothie that contains spinach, kale, banana, cherries, and a dollop of protein powder or Greek yogurt. To achieve the desirable consistency, incorporate a small amount of almond milk or coconut water. This smoothie is a powerful source of antioxidants, vitamins, and minerals that can help you start your day.

Breakfast Dishes That Are Beneficial For The Heart:

Construct a heart-healthy breakfast dish by combining cooked quinoa or oats with sliced fruits such as bananas, strawberries, and pears. Add a dollop of Greek yogurt, a scattering of almonds or seeds, and a drizzle of honey or maple syrup to add sweetness. This bowl is an ideal choice for promoting cardiac health, as it is abundant in fiber, antioxidants, and healthy lipids.

Egg Dishes That Are Effortless To Prepare:

Prepare a rapid and effortless egg dish by combining minced vegetables, such as bell peppers, spinach, and tomatoes, with scrambled eggs. To enhance the flavor, incorporate a small amount of cheese and seasonings. For a nutritious breakfast, pair it with avocado or whole-grain crostini. Eggs are an excellent source of protein and essential nutrients, including choline and vitamin D.

Waffles And Crepes Made From Whole Grains:

Substitute conventional crepes and waffles with whole-grain versions that are prepared with cereals or whole-wheat flour. Add pureed bananas or grated zucchini to the batter to enhance the sweetness and moisture without the need for additional sugar. For a nutritious and delectable breakfast, garnish with Greek yogurt, fresh fruit, or a drizzle of pure maple syrup.

Breakfast Options That Can Be Easily Consumed On The Go:

Combine oats or chia seeds with your preferred milk, yogurt, or fruit juice to create convenient breakfast options such as chia pudding or overnight oats. Incorporate flavorings such as vanilla extract, cocoa powder, or cinnamon, and refrigerate the mixture overnight. In the morning, simply take a jar or container and enjoy a nutritious and convenient meal on the go. These alternatives are adaptable and can be customized to accommodate your dietary requirements and personal preferences.

Lunch Recipes That Inspire Energy

Individuals with POTS syndrome must consume energizing lunch recipes to sustain consistent energy levels throughout the day.

Complex carbohydrates, lean proteins, healthy lipids, and an abundance of fruits and vegetables should be the primary components of these recipes. An example of an energizing supper is a quinoa salad topped with grilled chicken, avocado, spinach, and cherry tomatoes, drizzled with a lemon-olive oil vinaigrette. This meal offers a well-balanced composition of nutrients that can be consumed to maintain energy and prevent blood sugar fluctuations.

Salads Rich In Vitamins And Minerals

For patients with POTS syndrome, salads that are rich in vitamins and minerals are an excellent choice, as they provide essential nutrients without placing an undue burden on the digestive system. To optimize nutrient intake, choose a diverse array of colorful vegetables, including beets, cucumbers, carrots, bell peppers, and verdant greens.

For satiety, incorporate protein sources such as chickpeas, tofu, or grilled chicken. Spinach, kale, roasted sweet potatoes, quinoa, hazelnuts, and a citrus vinaigrette are all potential components of a nutrient-dense salad.

Lunch Ideas With Lean Protein

Individuals with POTS syndrome need to include lean protein in their meals to maintain muscle strength and stability. Skinless poultry, fish, tofu, legumes, and low-fat dairy products are all examples of lean protein sources. A brunch concept that is both straightforward and nutritious is grilled salmon, which is served with steamed asparagus and quinoa. Salmon is abundant in omega-3 fatty acids, which have anti-inflammatory properties and help maintain cardiac health. Quinoa is a comprehensive source of protein and fiber that provides long-lasting energy.

Hearty Soups And Stews

During the harsher months or when feeling unwell, hearty soups and stews are nutritious and comforting options for patients with POTS syndrome. To circumvent the excess sodium and additives that are frequently present in canned soups and stews, choose domestic alternatives that are prepared with fresh, whole ingredients.

A nutritious and satisfying broth that includes kidney beans, onions, celery, carrots, tomatoes, and seasonings is a hearty vegetable and bean soup. Furthermore, bone broth-based stews can offer collagen and other nutrients that are advantageous for digestion and joint health.

Sandwiches And Wraps That Are Quick And Simple To Prepare

Wraps and sandwiches are convenient options for hectic days or when on the go. They are quick and simple to prepare. Select whole grain wrappers or bread to enhance fiber and nutrient content, and assemble them with a blend of vegetables, lean protein, and healthy lipids. For instance, a turkey and avocado whole wheat wrap with lettuce, tomato, and mustard can be prepared in a matter of minutes and offers a harmonious combination of protein, healthy lipids, and carbohydrates to maintain energy levels throughout the day. For a vegetarian option, consider a sandwich made with grilled vegetables and humus on whole-grain bread, which is rich in fiber, vitamins, and minerals.

Recipes For Dinner That Satisfy

Focus on meals that are both delectable and beneficial for blood pressure regulation when preparing dinner for POTS (Postural Orthostatic Tachycardia Syndrome). To sustain consistent energy levels, choose lean proteins such as grilled poultry or fish, which can be coupled with complex carbohydrates like sweet potatoes or quinoa. Provide essential vitamins and minerals by incorporating a variety of colorful vegetables, such as broccoli, bell peppers, and spinach. For instance, a grilled salmon fillet served with roasted vegetables and quinoa is a nutritious and satisfying meal that aids in the management of POTS.

Concepts of a Balanced Dinner Plate: The construction of a balanced dinner plate for POTS entails the integration of a diverse array of food groups to ensure that essential nutrients are obtained while averting the onset of symptoms. To enhance fiber intake and facilitate digestion, it is recommended that you consume half of your plate with non-starchy vegetables, such as cucumbers, tomatoes, and verdant greens.

For muscle regeneration and satiety, allocate one-quarter of your plate to a lean protein source, such as tofu, turkey, or legumes. Finally, to prevent blood sugar surges and provide sustained energy, load the remaining quarter with whole grains such as brown rice or whole wheat pasta. For example, a well-rounded meal that assists in the management of POTS symptoms could consist of grilled chicken breast, steamed broccoli, and quinoa pilaf.

Main Courses that are Nutritious and Delicious: To prevent symptoms from exacerbating, the main courses for POTS should be flavorful, nutrient-dense, and simple to digest. Experiment with recipes that include lean proteins, such as turkey meatballs, broiled salmon, or tofu stir-fry, to provide muscle support and satiety without overtaxing the digestive system.

Enhance the flavor and facilitate nutrient assimilation by combining these proteins with a diverse array of seasonings, spices, and healthy fats, such as avocado or olive oil. For example, a turkey and vegetable stir-fry that is seasoned with ginger, garlic, and soy sauce and served over brown rice is a delectable and nutritious main course that is appropriate for POTS management.

Side Dishes Packed with Fiber and Nutrients: Side dishes are essential for a POTS-friendly diet, as they offer supplementary nutrients and fiber to promote digestion and overall health. To enhance fiber intake and induce regularity, opt for side dishes such as roasted root vegetables, steamed green beans, or a mixed salad containing carrots, tomatoes, and leafy greens.

To improve nutrient absorption and satiety, incorporate healthy lipids such as almonds, seeds, or avocado into vegetable dishes or salads. For example, a nutrient-rich and flavorful addition to any POTS-friendly entrée is a side of roasted sweet potatoes drizzled with olive oil and strewn with chopped almonds.

POTS-Friendly Pasta and Grain Dishes: Some modifications can be made to pasta and grain dishes to make them more supportive of symptom management when consumed on a POTS diet. To enhance fiber content and provide sustained energy without causing blood sugar surges, choose whole grain varieties such as brown rice, quinoa, or whole wheat pasta. Combine these grains with lean proteins, such as turkey meatballs, grilled chicken, or tofu, to create a nutritious meal that promotes satiety and muscle function.

To improve the taste of a dish without relying on processed ingredients or excessive sodium, experiment with condiments that are flavored with fresh herbs, vegetables, and olive oil.

For instance, a quinoa salad with grilled vegetables, chickpeas, and a lemon-herb vinaigrette provides a satisfying and invigorating alternative to a pasta and grain dish that is compatible with POTS.

CHAPTER FIVE

Snacks And Small Bites

It is essential to maintain consistent energy levels throughout the day when managing POTS syndrome. Opt for refreshment ideas that are simple to prepare, such as whole-grain crackers with humus or sliced fruits with nut butter. These offer a harmonious combination of protein, healthful lipids, and carbohydrates to maintain consistent blood sugar levels.

Consider portable munchies, including yogurt containers, trail mix, or pre-cut vegetables with dip, for on-the-go options. Smoothie bowls that are abundant in nutrients, such as spinach, berries, and Greek yogurt, provide a nutritious and pleasant refreshment option. Homemade dips and spreads that are prepared from avocado, Greek yogurt, or legumes are exceptional options for enhancing the flavor and nutritional value of munchies. Furthermore, energy-boosting snack bars that are composed of dried fruits, almonds, and oats can offer a rapid and convenient source of sustained energy in between meals.

Snacks That Are Effortless To Prepare:
Simplicity is paramount when preparing refreshments for individuals with POTS syndrome. For a gratifying combination of fiber and healthy lipids, consider slicing an apple and serving it with a tablespoon of almond butter.

Alternately, prepare a fast yogurt parfait by layering Greek yogurt with fresh berries and granola. These foods can be quickly assembled and offer a balanced combination of carbohydrates, protein, and fats to help regulate blood sugar levels and prevent energy declines.

Snacks That Can Be Transported:

It is crucial to have portable refreshments on hand during those hectic days when one is continuously on the move. For a convenient and energizing snack, it is advisable to bring a small container of dried fruits and assorted nuts. Another portable option that offers a well-balanced combination of carbohydrates and protein is rice cakes that are garnished with avocado or tuna salad.

In addition, a portable and fulfilling snack option that can be savored anywhere is provided by single-serve packets of nut butter paired with whole-grain crackers.

Smoothie Dishes That Are Abundant In Nutrients:

Smoothie dishes are a nutritious and delectable method of nourishing your body, particularly when you are combating POTS syndrome.

Combine spinach, banana, and almond milk to create a base that is rich in vitamins and minerals. Then, garnish your smoothie bowl with fresh fruits, nuts, and seeds to enhance the flavor and texture. In addition to being a refreshing and hydrating refreshment option that can help combat symptoms of fatigue and lightheadedness, smoothie bowls are also simple to customize to your preferences.

Dips And Condiments That Are Nutritious:

Dips and condiments can enhance the flavor and nutritional value of your munchies, thereby increasing their enjoyment and satisfaction. Choose homemade alternatives such as tzatziki, hummus, or guacamole, which are abundant in protein and healthful lipids.

These dips can be paired with sliced fruits, whole-grain crackers, or raw vegetables to create a balanced refreshment that can help prevent energy declines and stabilize blood sugar levels. To personalize the flavor of your sauces and spreads to your liking, experiment with a variety of herbs and seasonings.

Recipes For Beverages And Hydration

Hydration is essential for the management of POTS symptoms, as it assists in the regulation of blood volume and the maintenance of blood pressure. It is imperative to consume an ample amount of fluids throughout the day. Electrolyte-rich beverages can be particularly advantageous for preserving electrolyte equilibrium and averting dehydration.

Coconut water, citrus juices, and a sprinkle of sodium can be employed to prepare electrolyte-rich beverages at home. Herbal infusions can also aid in digestion, relaxation, and tension reduction, in addition to providing hydration benefits. A nutrient-rich energy boost can be achieved by consuming smoothies and beverages that are prepared with fruits, vegetables, and protein sources. To enhance the flavor of your hydration regimen, consider infusing water with cucumber slices, herbs, or citrus.

The Significance Of Hydration In POTS

Individuals with POTS need to maintain proper hydration, as they are more susceptible to dehydration as a result of reduced blood volume and increased fluid loss. Symptoms such as fatigue, vertigo, and lightheadedness may be exacerbated by dehydration.

Maintaining proper hydration levels can assist in the regulation of blood flow, the enhancement of circulation, and the maintenance of overall cardiovascular function.

Additionally, complications such as organ injury and syncope episodes can be prevented through consistent hydration.

Recipes For Drinks That Are Rich In Electrolytes

Individuals with POTS must consume electrolyte-rich beverages to replace the electrolytes that are lost through excessive perspiration and urine output. Coconut water, citrus fruits, and sea salt are all-natural constituents that can be used to formulate your electrolyte beverages.

A straightforward recipe entails the combination of coconut water, a sprinkle of salt, and a dash of lemon juice. This combination is essential for the maintenance of fluid homeostasis and the support of muscle function, as it contains potassium, sodium, and magnesium.

The Advantages Of Herbal Teas

Herbal infusions possess a variety of health-promoting properties in addition to providing hydration benefits. Certain herbal infusions can be beneficial for individuals with POTS, as they can ameliorate symptoms such as fatigue, vertigo, and bloating.

For example, peppermint tea can facilitate digestion and alleviate gastrointestinal distress, while chamomile tea may induce relaxation and alleviate tension. Ginger tea is another exceptional alternative for enhancing circulation and alleviating nausea.

Hydration can be improved and therapeutic effects can be augmented by incorporating herbal infusions into your daily regimen.

Smoothies and smoothies are convenient alternatives for individuals with POTS who may encounter challenges with meal preparation or have difficulty ingesting solid foods. Nutrient-rich constituents, including fruits, leafy greens, yogurt, and protein powder, may be included in these beverages.

Bananas, spinach, almond milk, and a sprinkle of protein powder comprise a straightforward smoothie that enhances vitality. The addition of nutritious lipids, such as avocado or nut butter, can further improve satiety and provide consistent energy throughout the day. By experimenting with various flavor combinations, you can personalize your smoothies to meet your nutritional requirements and taste preferences.

CHAPTER SIX

Strategies For Meal Planning And Preparation

It is essential to establish a weekly dietary plan to effectively manage the symptoms of POTS syndrome. Begin by compiling a list of foods that are high in potassium, low in sodium, and have a well-balanced ratio of carbohydrates and proteins. Incorporate a diverse selection of fruits, vegetables, lean proteins, and whole cereals into your diet.

During the week, it is possible to conserve energy and time by batch preparing and preserving meals. Prepare substantial quantities of soups, stews, or casseroles that can be preserved for future use. Some simple and quick meal prep ideas include preparing overnight oats for breakfast, bringing salads with grilled chicken and mixed greens for lunch, and roasting vegetables for a simple supper side. Meal preparation can be streamlined by organizing your kitchen for efficiency. Invest in time-saving kitchen devices such as a slow cooker or Instant Pot, label containers for leftovers, and keep frequently used ingredients within easy reach.

Sample meal plans that cater to a variety of needs may encompass vegetarian or vegan preferences, low-sodium diets, and specific calorie requirements. Investigate various menu combinations and recipes to determine which one is most suitable for your needs.

Nutrient-Rich Foods To Incorporate

Concentrate on the inclusion of nutrient-rich foods that can assist in the management of POTS symptoms when formulating your meal plan.

Choose foods that are high in potassium, such as bananas, sweet potatoes, spinach, and avocado, to assist in the regulation of blood pressure and fluid balance. Select lean proteins, such as chicken, turkey, fish, and tofu, to maintain energy levels and muscle strength.

To guarantee a comprehensive array of vitamins and minerals, it is recommended to consume an abundance of fruits and vegetables in a diversity of colors. Quinoa, brown rice, and oats are examples of whole grains that offer sustained energy without causing blood sugar surges.

Nuts, seeds, and olive oil are all sources of healthful fats that can also contribute to the maintenance of cardiac health and the enhancement of overall well-being.

Electrolyte And Hydration Balance

It is imperative to maintain hydration to effectively manage POTS syndrome, as dehydration can exacerbate symptoms such as fatigue and vertigo. Ensure that you consume an adequate amount of water throughout the day and consider incorporating electrolyte-rich beverages, such as coconut water or sports drinks, into your routine, particularly if you suffer from heat intolerance or excessive perspiration. It is crucial to closely monitor your fluid intake to prevent overhydration, which can dilute electrolyte levels.

In addition, the consumption of foods that are rich in electrolytes, such as bananas, oranges, yogurt, and leafy vegetables, can assist in the preservation of appropriate equilibrium.

Refrain from consuming excessive amounts of caffeine and alcohol, as they can exacerbate symptoms and contribute to dehydration.

Methods For Reducing Sodium

It is crucial to reduce sodium ingestion to manage POTS symptoms, as excessive salt consumption can result in increased blood pressure and fluid retention. Begin by reviewing food labels and selecting products with reduced sodium content whenever feasible. Cook meals from scratch with fresh ingredients and enhance the flavor of dishes with citrus juices, herbs, and seasonings in place of salt.

Before incorporating canned foods, such as legumes and vegetables, into recipes, rinse them to eliminate superfluous sodium. Reduce the consumption of processed and packaged foods, which are often high in sodium, and prioritize domestic alternatives whenever possible. Allow your taste receptors to acclimate to lower sodium levels over time by gradually reducing the amount of salt you add to meals.

Addressing Digestive Disorders

Bloating, constipation, or gastroparesis are common digestive symptoms among those with POTS syndrome. To alleviate these symptoms, it is recommended that you consume smaller, more frequent meals throughout the day, rather than larger, heavier meals that can exacerbate discomfort. Select readily digestible foods, such as cooked vegetables, lean proteins, and whole cereals, and chew your food thoroughly to facilitate digestion.

To prevent constipation and promote regular bowel movements, incorporate fiber-rich foods such as fruits, vegetables, legumes, and whole grains into your diet. To maintain digestive health, it is recommended that you consume water between meals and incorporate probiotic-rich foods such as yogurt, kefir, or sauerkraut.

Work with a healthcare provider or registered dietitian to create a personalized eating plan that accommodates your specific dietary restrictions or intolerances while simultaneously managing the symptoms of POTS.

CHAPTER SEVEN

Seven Days Meal Plan, Recipes, Ingredients, And Detailed Preparatory Guidelines For Pots Syndrome

DAY ONE:

• Breakfast:

o Recipe: Breakfast Bowl with Quinoa

o. **INGREDIENTS**:

☐ Fresh vegetables

☐ Cherry tomatoes

☐ Eggs

☐ Olive oil

☐ Pepper and salt

• *PREPARATION:*

1. Prepare the quinoa by the instructions provided in the package.

2. Sauté cherry tomatoes and spinach in olive oil.

3. Fry or poach eggs.

4. Combine sautéed vegetables, cooked quinoa, sliced avocado, and eggs in a basin. Add salt and pepper to taste.

Lunch:

Grilled Chicken Salad Recipe

INGREDIENTS:

☐ Chicken breast

☐ Greens blended

Watermelon

☐ Bell peppers

☐ Red onion

☐ Olive oil

☐ Balsamic vinegar

☐ Pepper and salt

PREPARATION:

Grill the chicken breast until it is fully cooked, then season it with salt and pepper.

1. Chop red onion, bell peppers, cucumber, and assorted greens.

2. Toss the salad ingredients with the sliced seared chicken.

3. Season with salt and pepper to flavor, then drizzle with olive oil and balsamic vinegar.

INGREDIENTS:

☐ Fillets of salmon

☐ Fresh herbs, including thyme, chives, and parsley

☐ Garlic

☐ Olive oil

☐ Pepper and salt

PREPARATION:

Preheat the oven to 375°F (190°C).

1. Arrange the salmon fillets on a baking sheet that has been lined with parchment paper.

2. Drizzle with lemon juice and olive oil, and then garnish with minced garlic, diced herbs, salt, and pepper.

3. Bake the salmon for 12-15 minutes or until it is fully cooked.

DAY TWO:

• Breakfast:

o Recipe: Berry Smoothie Bowl

o. **INGREDIENTS**:

☐ Strawberry, blueberry, and raspberry mixture

☐ Banana

☐ Greek yogurt

Honey

☐ Granola

• ***PREPARATION:***

1. Combine Greek yogurt, banana, and assorted berries in a blender until the mixture is homogeneous.

2. Transfer to a dish.

3. Add granola and a drizzle of honey to the top.

Lunch:

Recipe: Turkey and Avocado Wrap

INGREDIENTS:

• Wrap made from whole grain

Pts Turkey breast, sliced

Onions

Carrot

☐ Hummus

PREPARATION:

Arrange the bundle made from whole grain.

1. Distribute the hummus uniformly across the wrap.

2. Sliced turkey breast, avocado, lettuce, and tomato are arranged in a layer.

3. Twist the roll securely and then cut it in half.

Dinner:

Vegetarian Stir-Fry Recipe

INGREDIENTS:

☐ Tofu

The following vegetables are included in the mixture: broccoli, carrots, snap peas, and bell peppers.

☐ Soy sauce

☐ Garlic

Pts Sesame oil

☐ Rice is optional.

PREPARATION:

The tofu should be pressed to remove any superfluous moisture, and then it should be cut into cubes.

1. Heat sesame oil in a large skillet or griddle over medium heat.

2. Stir-fry minced garlic and ginger until they are aromatic.

3. Stir-fry the assorted vegetables and tofu until the vegetables are tender-crisp.

4. Add soy sauce to your liking.

5. If preferred, serve with rice.

THIRD DAY:

• Breakfast:

o Recipe: Banana and Almond Butter Oatmeal

o. **INGREDIENTS**:

☐ Rolled oats

☐ Almond milk

☐ Almond butter

☐ Banana

Honey

• PREPARATION:

1. Use almond milk to prepare rolled cereals according to the instructions on the container.

2. Cut the banana into slices.

3. Add almond butter and stir until thoroughly combined.

4. Add a drizzle of honey and a sliced banana to the top.

INGREDIENTS:

Beans

☐ Carrots

☐ Corn

☐ One onion

☐ Garlic

☐ Vegetable bouillon

☐ Bay fronds

☐ Olive oil

☐ Pepper and salt

PREPARATION:

In a sizable skillet, heat olive oil over medium heat.

1. Sauté minced onion, carrots, celery, and garlic until they are tender.

2. Incorporate bay leaves, vegetable bouillon, and lentils.

3. Bring the mixture to a boil, then reduce the heat and allow it to simmer until the lentils are soft.

4. Adjust the salt and pepper to taste.

INGREDIENTS:

☐ Chicken legs

☐ Sweet potatoes

☐ Olive oil

☐ Paprika

Cucumber

☐ Garlic granules

☐ Pepper and salt

PREPARATION:

. Preheat the oven to 400°F (200°C).

1. Season chicken thighs with paprika, cumin, garlic powder, salt, and pepper after rubbing them with olive oil.

2. Dice sweet potatoes after they have been peeled.

3. Arrange sweet potatoes and chicken thighs on a baking sheet that has been lined with parchment paper.

4. Bake for 25-30 minutes or until the sweet potatoes are tender and the chicken is fully cooked.

DAY FOUR:

• Breakfast:

o Recipe: Greek Yogurt Parfait

o. **INGREDIENTS**:

☐ Greek yogurt

☐ Granola

☐ A combination of fruit

Honey

• *PREPARATION:*

1. Combine Greek yogurt, granola, and a variety of berries in a basin or glass.

2. Use honey to drizzle.

Lunch:

Recipe: Quinoa Salad with Feta and Chickpeas

INGREDIENTS:

☐ Chickpeas

Watermelon

☐ Cherry tomatoes

☐ Red onion

☐ Feta cheese

☐ Olive oil

☐ Pepper and salt

PREPARATION:

Prepare the quinoa according to the instructions provided on the package.

1. Chickpeas should be rinsed and drained.

2. Cut cucumber, cherry tomatoes, and red onion into small pieces.

3. Combine cooked quinoa, lentils, chopped vegetables, crumbled feta cheese, lemon juice, and olive oil in a large basin.

4. Adjust the salt and pepper to taste.

Dinner:

Salmon and asparagus foil packets are the recipe.

INGREDIENTS:

☐ Fillets of salmon

Pts Asparagus spears

☐ Garlic

☐ Olive oil

☐ Pepper and salt

PREPARATION:

Preheat the oven to 400°F (200°C).

1. Arrange salmon fillets on aluminum foil.

2. Assemble asparagus segments around the salmon.

3. Apply a mixture of olive oil, lemon juice, minced garlic, salt, and pepper.

4. Create containers by folding the foil.

5. Bake for 15-20 minutes or until the asparagus is tender and the salmon is fully cooked.

DAY FIVE:

• Breakfast:

o Spinach and Mushroom Omelette Recipe

o. **INGREDIENTS**:

☐ Eggs

☐ Spinach

☐ Mushrooms

☐ One onion

☐ Olive oil

☐ Pepper and salt

• *PREPARATION:*

1. In a skillet, heat olive oil over medium heat.

2. Sauté minced onion and cut mushrooms until they are tender.

3. Add spinach and simmer until it is wilted.

4. Pour the eggs into the skillet after whisking them in a basin.

5. Fold the omelet in half after cooking until it is fully set. Add salt and pepper to taste.

Lunch:

Turkey and Vegetable Soup Recipe

INGREDIENTS:

☐ Turkey breast

☐ Carrots

☐ Corn

☐ One onion

☐ Garlic

☐ Chicken bouillon

☐ Bay fronds

☐ Olive oil

☐ Pepper and salt

PREPARATION:

In a sizable skillet, heat olive oil over medium heat.

1. Sauté minced onion, carrots, celery, and garlic until they are tender.

2. Add the diced turkey breast and sauté until it is browned.

3. Add bay leaves, pour in chicken broth, and bring to a simmer.

4. Allow the mixture to simmer for 20-25 minutes until the flavors have merged and the turkey is fully cooked. Adjust the salt and pepper to taste.

Dinner:

Beef and Broccoli Stir-Fry Recipe

INGREDIENTS:

Beef tenderloin

☐ Broccoli flowers

☐ Soy sauce

☐ Garlic

Garlic

Pts Sesame oil

☐ Rice is optional.

PREPARATION:

Thinly slice beef sirloin against the grain.

1. Heat sesame oil in a large skillet or griddle over medium heat.

2. Stir-fry minced garlic and ginger until they are aromatic.

3. Add the sliced beef and sauté until it is browned.

4. Stir-fry broccoli florets and soy sauce until the broccoli is tender-crisp.

5. If preferred, serve with rice.

DAY SIX:

o. **INGREDIENTS**:

☐ Chia seeds

☐ Almond milk

Honey

Coffee extract

☐ A combination of fruit

• *PREPARATION:*

1. In a basin or container, combine almond milk, honey, vanilla extract, and chia seeds.

2. Stir the mixture thoroughly, cover it, and place it in the refrigerator for the night.

3. Top with a mixture of berries.

Caprese Salad Recipe

INGREDIENTS:

• Fresh mozzarella

Carrot

☐ Basil, fresh

☐ Balsamic vinegar

☐ Olive oil

☐ Pepper and salt

PREPARATION:

Fresh mozzarella and tomato should be sliced.

1. Alternately arrange slices of mozzarella, tomato, and fresh basil leaves on a plate.

2. Apply a mixture of olive oil and balsamic vinegar to the dish.

3. Add salt and pepper to your liking.

Dinner:

Shrimp and Zucchini Noodles Recipe

INGREDIENTS:

Ramp

☐ Penne

☐ Garlic

☐ Olive oil

Clementine

☐ Peppercorns

☐ Pepper and salt

PREPARATION:

Spiralize zucchini to create strands.

1. In a skillet, heat olive oil over medium heat.

2. Add minced garlic and red pepper flakes, and sauté until the mixture is aromatic.

3. Add the shrimp and sauté until they are opaque and pink.

4. Add zucchini noodles and simmer until they are soft.

5. Season the dish with salt and pepper and squeeze lemon juice over it.

SEVENTH DAY:

• Breakfast:

o Recipe: Breakfast Burrito

o. **INGREDIENTS**:

☐ Whole grain tortilla

☐ Black legumes

☐ Mexican rice

☐ Cheddar cheese

• *PREPARATION:*

1. Heat the tortilla in a skillet or microwave.

2. Stuff with shredded cheddar cheese, salsa, sliced avocado, black beans, and scrambled eggs.

3. Tightly roll and serve.

Tuna Salad Lettuce Wraps Recipe

INGREDIENTS:

☐ Tuna canned

☐ Corn

☐ Red onion

☐ Greek yogurt

☐ Dijon mustard

• Lettuce leaves

☐ Pepper and salt

PREPARATION:

1. Incorporate diced celery, red onion, Greek yogurt, Dijon mustard, and lemon juice. Combine thoroughly.

2. Add salt and pepper to your liking.

3. Spoon tuna salad into lettuce leaves and enclose them.

INGREDIENTS:

☐ Black legumes

☐ Kidney legumes

☐ Bell peppers

☐ One onion

☐ Garlic

Dices tomatoes

- Tomato juice

• Chili powder

Cucumber

☐ Paprika

☐ Olive oil

☐ Pepper and salt

PREPARATION:

In a sizable skillet, heat olive oil over medium heat.

1. Sauté garlic, bell peppers, and onion until they are tender.

2. Stir in minced tomatoes, tomato paste, black beans, kidney beans, chile powder, cumin, paprika, salt, and pepper.

3. Bring the mixture to a simmer and cook for 20-25 minutes, whisking intermittently.

4. Serve at a high temperature.

Snacks:

- A mixture of legumes

- Hummus with carrot spears

- Greek yogurt with hazelnuts and honey

- Cakes made with rice and almond butter

- Peanut butter on apple wedges

Juice:

- Green juice

o. **INGREDIENTS**:

Spinach

Watermelon

Corn

Green apples

Garlic

• PREPARATION:

1. Utilize an extractor to extract all ingredients.

2. Mix thoroughly and serve over ice.

Please feel free to modify the recipes and ingredients to suit your dietary restrictions and preferences. I hope you enjoy your meals!

CHAPTER EIGHT

Seven Desserts Procedural Recipes For Pots Syndrome And Guidelines

Postural Orthostatic Tachycardia Syndrome (POTS) can have a substantial impact on daily life, including dietary decisions. A high-sodium diet and sufficient hydration are frequently necessary for the management of POTS. Although desserts may not be the first item that comes to mind for individuals following a high-sodium diet, there are methods to savor sweet treats while still adhering to dietary requirements.

Seven simple confection recipes that are appropriate for patients with POTS are presented below, with an emphasis on ingredients that adhere to the essential dietary guidelines.

INGREDIENTS:

- One cup of butter

- Two cups of sugar

- Four large eggs

- One cup of all-purpose flour

- One cup of unadulterated cocoa powder

- 1/2 teaspoon of baking powder

- One teaspoon of vanilla extract

- One-half teaspoon of salt

- One cup of caramel sauce

- Flakes of sea salt

STEPS:

1. Preheat the oven to 350°F (175°C). Grease a pastry tin that measures 9 inches by 13 inches.

2. Melt butter in a medium saucepan. Stir in sugar, eggs, and vanilla after removing from heat.

3. Combine the flour, cocoa powder, baking powder, and salt by sifting them. Then, incorporate the mixture into the butter.

4. Distribute half of the batter evenly across the prepared pan. Swirl the batter with a knife after drizzling half of the caramel sauce over it.

5. Pour the remaining batter over the caramel and repeat the process with the remaining caramel sauce.

6. Bake for 25 to 30 minutes. After baking, sprinkle sea salt crystals over the top.

INGREDIENTS:

• Two mature avocados

• 1/4 cup of Nutella

• One cup of milk (or a dairy substitute)

• One tablespoon of honey

• 1/4 teaspoon of salt

• Ice crystals

STEPS:

1. In a processor, combine bananas, Nutella, milk, honey, and salt.

2. Blend in ice crystals until the mixture is smooth.

3. Serve immediately.

INGREDIENTS:

• 1/2 cup of chia seeds

• Two glasses of milk (or a dairy substitute)

• One teaspoon of vanilla extract

• Two tablespoons of honey

• 1/4 teaspoon of salt

• Fresh cherries for garnish

STEPS:

1. Combine chia seeds, milk, vanilla extract, honey, and salt in a basin.

2. Agitate the mixture thoroughly and allow it to settle for 10 minutes. Subsequently, agitate the mixture once more to prevent clumping.

3. Cover and refrigerate for a minimum of four hours or overnight.

4. Before serving, garnish with fresh cherries.

4. CHOCOLATE CHIP COOKIES WITH A SALTY FLAVOR

INGREDIENTS:

- 1 cup of clarified butter

- One cup of sugar

- One cup of brown sugar

- Two large embryos

- Two tablespoons of vanilla extract

- Three cups of all-purpose flour

- One teaspoon of baking soda

- 1/2 teaspoon of baking powder

• One-half teaspoon of salt

• Two cups of chocolate chunks

• Flakes of sea salt

STEPS:

1. Preheat the oven to 350°F (175°C). Line baking sheets with parchment paper.

2. Combine the butter and sugars until they are light and frothy. Combine vanilla and eggs; beat thoroughly.

3. In an additional container, combine salt, baking powder, baking soda, and flour. The butter mixture should be gradually added to.

4. Add chocolate chunks and mix thoroughly.

5. Drop the mixture onto the baking trays in rounded spoonfuls. Add sea salt granules to the dish.

6. Bake for 10-12 minutes or until the surface is a rich golden color.

INGREDIENTS:

• Two cups of Greek yogurt

• 1/4 cup of honey

• 1/4 cup of chopped almonds

• 1/4 teaspoon of salt

STEPS:

1. Distribute Greek yogurt among serving dishes.

2. Apply honey to the yogurt.

3. Sprinkle salt and sliced hazelnuts on top.

4. Serve immediately.

INGREDIENTS:

• Two pints of heavy cream

• One cup of whole milk

• One cup of sugar

• One-half cup of caramel sauce

• One teaspoon of vanilla extract

• 1/4 teaspoon of sea salt

STEPS:

1. Heat the cream, milk, and sugar in a medium saucepan until the sugar has dissolved.

2. Stir in the caramel sauce, vanilla extract, and sea salt after removing from the flame.

3. Allow the mixture to settle before churning it to an ice cream maker by the manufacturer's instructions.

4. Transfer the mixture to a container and freeze until it is solid.

7. ALMOND BARK WITH SALTED CHOCOLATE FLAVOR

INGREDIENTS:

• 12 ounces of grated dark chocolate

• 1 cup of toasted and sliced almonds

• One-half teaspoon of sea salt

STEPS:

1. Melt chocolate in a microwave or double boiler until it is smooth.

2. Stir in sea salt and pistachios.

3. Transfer the mixture to a baking sheet that has been lined with parchment paper.

4. After allowing it to settle completely, it should be broken into fragments.

Pots-Friendly Dessert Guidelines

1. Salt: When feasible, incorporate sea salt to satisfy sodium requirements and improve flavor.

2. Hydration: Incorporate delicacies such as chia seed pudding and smoothies to increase fluid intake.

3. Moderation: Consume desserts in moderation, ensuring that they are balanced with nutrient-dense meals.

4. Nutritious Ingredients: Incorporate ingredients that offer supplementary nutritional advantages, such as almonds, Greek yogurt, and fresh fruits.

5. Customizable: Recipes can be modified to accommodate dietary preferences or restrictions, such as the use of gluten-free flour or dairy alternatives.

While taking into account the dietary requirements of patients with POTS, these delicacies can offer a delicious respite. With careful ingredient selection and preparation techniques, it is feasible to relish food, including desserts.

CHAPTER NINE

Seven Smoothies Procedural Recipes For Pots Syndrome And Guidelines

1. Hydration: Patients with POTS frequently require an increase in their fluid intake. Aim for fruits and vegetables that are high in water content.

2. Electrolytes: Incorporate ingredients that are high in electrolytes, such as bananas, coconut water, and verdant vegetables.

3. Sustained Energy: Guarantee that your diet contains a balanced combination of carbohydrates, proteins, and healthy lipids.

4. Low Sugar: To prevent blood sugar surges, choose low-glycemic produce.

5. Digestive Ease: Select ingredients that are readily digestible to prevent gastrointestinal discomfort.

6. Anti-inflammatory: Incorporate anti-inflammatory ingredients, including turmeric, ginger, and fruit.

7. Portion Control: Consuming smaller, more frequent meals can be more effective in alleviating symptoms than consuming larger portions.

RECIPE 1: HYDRATION HERO

INGREDIENTS:

• One cup of coconut water

• One cucumber, sliced

• 1 cup of sliced cantaloupe

• One tablespoon of chia seeds

• The juice of one citrus

• Ice crystals

STEPS:

1. Combine lime juice, cucumber, melons, and coconut water in a blender.

2. Blend until the mixture is uniform.

3. Incorporate chia seeds and blend briefly once more.

4. Please serve immediately over ice.

RECIPE 2: ELECTROLYTE ENERGIZER

INGREDIENTS:

• One banana

• One cup of spinach

• One cup of almond milk

• One tablespoon of almond butter

• One tablespoon of honey

• One teaspoon of flaxseed

STEPS:

1. In a Vitamix, combine almond milk, almond butter, honey, spinach, and a banana.

2. Blend until the mixture is smooth and velvety.

3. Add flaxseed and pulverize a few times.

4. Pour the beverage into a glass and savor it.

RECIPE 3: ECO-FRIENDLY INGREDIENTS

INGREDIENTS:

• One cup of kale

• One green apple, cored and sliced

• One-half of an avocado

• One cup of coconut water

• One teaspoonful of lemon juice

• Ice crystals

STEPS:

1. Combine kale, green apple, avocado, coconut water, and lemon juice in a blender.

2. Blend until the mixture is velvety and smooth.

3. Incorporate ice crystals and blend once more to achieve the desired consistency.

4. Chill before serving.

RECIPE 4: BERRY BLISS

INGREDIENTS:

• One cup of a combination of berries, including raspberries, blueberries, and strawberries

• One-half cup of Greek yogurt

• One cup of strained almond milk

• One tablespoon of chia seeds

• One teaspoon of honey (optional)

STEPS:

1. Blend almond milk, Greek yogurt, and assorted berries in a blender.

2. Blend until the mixture is homogeneous and well-integrated.

3. Incorporate chia seeds and blend briefly once more.

4. If preferred, add honey to the mixture.

5. Serve immediately.

RECIPE 5: TROPICAL TURMERIC

INGREDIENTS:

• One cup of pineapple slices

• Chopped half of a mango

• One cup of coconut milk

• 1/2 teaspoon of turmeric powder

• 1 teaspoon of minced ginger

• Ice crystals

STEPS:

1. Incorporate pineapple, mango, coconut milk, turmeric, and ginger into a Vitamix.

2. Blend until the mixture is entirely homogeneous.

3. Incorporate ice crystals and blend once more to achieve the desired consistency.

4. Pour the mixture into a glass and relish the tropical flavor.

INGREDIENTS:

• One spoonful of vanilla protein powder

• One banana

• 1/2 cup of oats

• One tablespoon of peanut butter

• One cup of almond milk

• One tablespoon of honey

STEPS:

1. In a blender, combine almond milk, honey, peanut butter, banana, oats, and protein powder.

2. Blend until the mixture is viscous and smooth.

3. If the consistency is excessively viscous, incorporate an additional tablespoon of almond milk.

4. Serve in a tall glass.

INGREDIENTS:

• One cup of blueberries

• One-half cup of Greek yogurt

• 1/2 teaspoon of turmeric powder

• One teaspoon of honey

• One cup of strained almond milk

• One teaspoon of cinnamon

STEPS:

1. Combine blueberries, Greek yogurt, turmeric, honey, almond milk, and cinnamon in a Vitamix.

2. Blend until the mixture is well-combined and creamy.

3. If necessary, increase the flavor by incorporating additional honey.

4. For an invigorating refreshment, serve chilled.

Optimal Smoothie Experience Tips

• Prepare in advance: Prepare the ingredients in advance and store them in freezer containers for fast blending.

• Adjust Consistency: Adjust the consistency of your smoothies by adjusting the amount of liquid added.

• Flavor Boost: Improve the flavor of the product by incorporating natural extracts such as almond or vanilla.

• Smoothie Bowls: For a crunchy texture, pour viscous smoothies into bowls and garnish with nuts, seeds, or fresh fruits.

By maintaining hydration, harmonizing electrolytes, and providing a consistent source of energy, the incorporation of these nutrient-rich smoothies into your diet can assist in the management of POTS symptoms. Experiment with these recipes and do not hesitate to modify the ingredients to accommodate your nutritional requirements and personal preferences.

Healthy Living With POTS Syndrome: Lifestyle Suggestions

To effectively manage symptoms, it is necessary to adopt a healthy lifestyle while living with Postural Orthostatic Tachycardia Syndrome (POTS). The following are indispensable lifestyle recommendations:

Safely incorporating exercise: Begin with low-impact activities, such as cycling or swimming, and progressively increase the intensity.

Strive to enhance blood flow through consistent, moderate movements that do not induce symptoms. Monitor your symptoms and heart rate to establish the appropriate equilibrium.

Stress management strategies: Engage in relaxation techniques, including deep breathing, meditation, or yoga, to alleviate stress. Identify stress triggers and devise effective coping strategies to manage them. Seek additional assistance through counseling or support groups.

Importance of sleep and rest: Establish a soothing twilight routine and adhere to a consistent sleep schedule to prioritize quality sleep. Maintain a slumber environment that is conducive to relaxation, such as maintaining a dark and silent space. To prevent exhaustion, it is important to listen to your body and take pauses as required throughout the day.

Establishing a supportive network: Surround yourself with healthcare professionals, family members, and companions who are empathetic and can provide you with support and motivation. Provide them with information regarding POTS to facilitate their comprehension of your condition. Additionally, valuable connections and advice can be obtained by participating in local or online support groups.

Monitoring and monitoring your progress: Maintain a symptom journal to track the efficacy of treatment strategies, triggers, and fluctuations in symptoms. Utilize wearable devices or applications to monitor sleep patterns, activity levels, and pulse rate. Review your progress with your healthcare team regularly to ensure that your treatment plans are adjusted as needed.

Conclusion

The significance of targeted nutritional strategies to effectively manage symptoms is underscored by the conclusion on the diet for Postural Orthostatic Tachycardia Syndrome (POTS). To relieve orthostatic intolerance, a POTS-friendly diet typically involves an increase in fluid and sodium intake, which increases blood volume. Hydration is essential, with frequently recommended intakes of 2-3 liters of water per day. A higher sodium intake, approximately 3,000 to 10,000 milligrams per day, can aid in the retention of fluids and the restoration of blood pressure stability.

To prevent blood sugar surges and maintain consistent energy levels, it is crucial to consume meals that are well-balanced and contain complex carbohydrates, protein, and fiber. A priority should be given to foods such as fruits, vegetables, whole cereals, and lean proteins. It is advisable to consume small, frequent meals rather than large meals, as the latter can exacerbate symptoms such as fatigue and lightheadedness.

Furthermore, it is advisable to refrain from consuming common triggers, such as caffeine and alcohol, as they can exacerbate POTS symptoms and lead to dehydration. A gluten-free or anti-inflammatory diet may be advantageous for certain individuals; however, these adjustments should be tailored to the specific triggers and intolerances of the individual.

In general, dietary management, in conjunction with medical treatment and lifestyle modifications, is essential for the enhancement of the quality of life of POTS patients by assisting in the stabilization of blood pressure and the reduction of symptom severity.

THE END